LIVE A REFLUX FREE LIFE

FREE LIFE

A Guide to Acid Reflux Diet

BY

BILL HILLON

Legal & Disclaimer

The content or information contained in this book is not designed to replace or take the place of any form of medical or professional advice; and is not meant to replace the need for independent medical, financial, legal or other professional advice or services, as may be required. The content or information in this book has been provided for educational and entertainment purposes only.

The content or information contained in this book is from sources deemed reliable, and it is accurate to the best of the author's knowledge, information and belief. However, the author cannot guarantee its accuracy and validity and cannot be held liable for any errors and/or omissions. Further changes are periodically made to this book as and when needed. Where appropriate and necessary, you must consult a professional (including but not limited to your doctor, attorney, financial advisor or such other professional advisor) before using

Table of Contents

INTRODUCTION

It is estimated that about 4 to 10 percent of adults show signs and symptoms of acid reflux daily. The symptoms are prevalent among those living in Western countries with up to 30 percent of adults from these countries weekly. Due to our individual differences, it's quite important that we strike the right balance between acid reflux drugs, diet and lifestyle modifications. For instance, acid reflux treatment plan may include eating an acid reflux diet, yoga, exercise, acupuncture, weight loss and alternative remedies.

If the acid reflux persists, it will eventually lead to the eroding of the esophagus wall and other complications. Severe untreated cases can lead to tissue scarring and formation of esophageal cancer.

The following chapters will give you enough information on acid reflux. They will show how you can effectively manage it without taking the fun out of your life. Ensure you don't just skim through this book but you take your time to carefully study every chapter in this book.

Happy reading!

CHAPTER ONE

WHAT IS ACID REFLUX AND ITS CAUSES?

Acid reflux, also known as heartburn, results from the regurgitation of digestive juices from the stomach back to the esophagus. These digestive juices are acidic in nature thereby causing a burning sensation and make you feel like a fire is in your throat or chest. It's a common belief that acid reflux is caused by eating foods that are high in acid content, thereby, producing too much acid in the stomach to cause acid reflux. However, this is not entirely true as poor digestion and low stomach acid are the more likely causes.

Acid reflux has similar symptoms to that of GERD, although GERD symptoms could be more severe. The basic cause of acid reflux is lack of proper functioning of the lower esophageal sphincter

(LES). The LES functions like a cover as it prevents acid from reverse flow into the esophagus. The stomach wall is being protected from the acid burning sensation while the esophagus does not, since its wall is not thickened like that of the stomach.

If you are experiencing this anomaly in digestion, note that this won't go away overnight by simply making a diet change and lifestyle changes, but with a consistent approach, you will definitely find the relief you crave for.

CHAPTER TWO

ACID REFLUX SYMPTOMS, CAUSES AND RISK FACTORS

There are certain foods that irritate the digestive system and leads to acid reflux. Some of these food includes processed foods, fried foods, sugary snacks, and refined oils.

For those suffering from acid reflux, symptoms include:

- Chest pains and burning sensations
- Bitter taste in your mouth
- Difficulty sleeping at night
- Gum irritation
- Bad breath
- Coughing or choking at midnight
- Dry mouth
- Stomach bloating after meals

- Sometimes nausea, loss of appetite and difficulty in eating many foods.

While there are various reasons why people develop these digestive disorders, acid reflux major causes which lead to painful symptoms for many people include:

- Rushing your food without proper chewing and not allowing adequate time for digestion. We are in a jet age and our society has been transformed into a fast-paced one, which is believed to be one of the most common causes of acid reflux.
- Overeating

This exerts so much pressure on the digestive system and it affects the stomach. Instead of spacing your meal and binge eating, you would curb acid reflux by electing to eat only 1-2 big meals per day.

- Obesity and being overweight
- Older age

This affects acid production

- History of hiatal hernias
- Pregnancy

Certain medications such as asthma, cardiac, arthritis, blood pressure drugs and repeat antibiotics also increase your chances of having acid reflux.

Chronic stress, deficiencies in certain nutrients, alcohol, smoking, and high caffeine can also predispose one to acid reflux.

CHAPTER THREE

NATURAL REMEDIES FOR ACID REFLUX

We often treat acid reflux with drugs to ameliorate the pain. These drugs are to prevent either the symptoms of acid reflux or when the symptoms are getting obvious. Some medicines recommended for treating acid reflux symptoms include Antacids and H2RAs. For those that have suffered from acid reflux symptoms in the past, they may have resulted in using some pills such as antacids, Tagamet, Pepcid AC, Zantac 75, and others.

Research has shown that use of drugs to cure the symptoms of acid reflux could lead to certain adverse effects such as poor digestion, depression, anemia, irritation of the bowel and fatigue. Long-term use of drugs like proton pump inhibitors or antacid could increase the chances of contracting infections such as C. difficile. This could further degenerate into complications such as diarrhea, bleeding ulcers and sore intestines. The old ones are at the greatest risk of the side effects from PPI as it could lead to certain chronic medical conditions.

The problems associated with conventional treatments have led to seeking home remedies for acid reflux. The natural remedies include supplements and essential oils.

1. Supplements for Acid Reflux Symptoms

Besides eating a healthy diet to reduce the acid reflux symptoms, it's also important to include natural supplements to your diet.

- Digestive Enzymes

Make use of digestive enzymes at the start of each meal by taking a capsule or two. They function to help digest and properly absorb nutrients.

- Probiotics

Probiotics add healthy bacteria to our guts. You will need about 25–50 billion units of it daily. It balances your digestive tract and eliminates bad bacteria responsible for indigestion, poor nutrients absorption and leaky guts.

- HCl with Pepsin

Prior to each meal, you should take one 650 mg of this pill. You could also take it along with other pills that will help to manage the uncomfortable symptoms at bay.

- Chamomile tea

Before going to bed at night, you should take one cup of chamomile tea alongside raw honey. Chamomile tea supports healthy functioning of the digestive tract as well as helping to reduce inflammation.

- Ginger tea

Ginger tea is a good remedy for acid reflux symptoms especially when it is just starting. Simply boil for 10 minutes one-inch size of ginger in 10 ounces of water sweetened with honey. You can take it either after dinner or just before going to bed. Ginger is widely used by many for digestive support. Instead of fresh ginger, you could still do with a ginger supplement in capsule form.

- Pawpaw leaf tea

Pawpaw contains an enzyme known as Papain. This enzyme aids digestion through the breaking down of proteins. Organic pawpaw tea is a good alternative in the absence of fresh organic, non-GMO pawpaw leaf. Take one cup of pawpaw once you start feeling the acid reflux symptoms before going to bed.

- Magnesium supplement

Acid reflux can be effectively treated using magnesium as it helps in the proper functioning of the sphincter. Simply take 400mg of magnesium complex supplement twice daily.

- L-Glutamine

L-Glutamine is known to help heal leaky guts. Take 5g of glutamine powder with meals twice daily.

- Melatonin

Several types of research have shown that most people suffering from acid reflux have a low melatonin level. Therefore, if it's been added to the body, it will boost your ability to cope with acid reflux. Simply take 6mg each evening.

2. Essential Oils

Lemon and lemon essential oil can help put in check acid reflux in some acid reflux patients.

Although it doesn't work for everyone as not everyone responds to this in the same way. Try mixing lemon juice with water with a slice of fresh ginger daily. Lemon essential oil can also be added to water and your drink.

3. Change the Way You Eat & Chew

Do not overeat – allow your food to digest properly by eating smaller meals. Overeating and large meals put the sphincter in too much pressure and it can result in regurgitation of undigested foods along with acid in the stomach.

Desist from eating three hours before retiring into bed. Give your stomach enough time to digest the foods while you sip a herbal tea sweetened with honey for relief digestive upset.

Thoroughly chew your meal—nowadays most people are guilty of not chewing their food enough; note that digestion starts in the mouth! Because when you take your time to chew your food properly, more salivary amylase is released.

This further breaks down the food and makes it easier for your stomach to digest them.

Ensure you wear comfortable cloth after eating — do not wear clothes that are too tight-fitted during mealtime and immediately after mealtime. This can further aggravate the symptoms and pain.

4. Other Lifestyle Changes & Tips

You need a multi-prong approach to cure acid reflux. Making wholesale lifestyle changes such as eating a healthy diet and balanced diet, avoiding trigger foods and taking the right supplements can all play important roles in reducing its symptoms.

To find relief from these acid reflux symptoms, you need to undergo certain lifestyle changes and improve your diet. These changes could be as simple as changing your sleeping pattern and stress management.

CHAPTER FOUR
THE ACID REFLUX DIET

One of the most prevalent causes of acid reflux is poorly processed diet. Overeating of processed food is also a cause as you have the tendency to neglect healthy eating practice when you do overeat. While we all have different stomach types and different reactions to foods, we are all sensitive to certain foods that trigger acid reflux. You must, therefore, be ready to first cut out those "consistent offenders" from your diet.

GMO foods need to be identified and eradicated from our meals in order for you to enjoy a soothing relief from pain and a good digestive health. Increase your fiber consumption, eat more of probiotic foods as it helps to support healthy bacteria, reduce grains, and eat high quality protein to protect the digestive tract. Aside from reducing acid reflux symptoms, making wholesale changes in your diet also helps to reduce the risk of obesity and complications from chronic diseases.

Foods That Fight Acid Reflux

- Oatmeal

This is known as one of the best breakfast, and the snack is recommended by the reflux diet any time of the day. Even if you make instant oatmeal with raisins, the oatmeal absorbs the acidity of the raisins.

- Ginger

Ginger is part of the best foods for acid reflux. They used this as an anti-inflammatory and as a treatment for gastrointestinal condition throughout in history. Ginger root is easy to peel and diced. You can use this when cooking; you should add it to smoothies, snack on ginger chews or sip ginger tea.

- Aloe Vera

Aloe Vera is well known as a natural healing agent and it seems to treat acid reflux. This can be planted in one's garden, but the leaves and liquid can be sold separately in grocery stores. Aloe Vera can play the role as a thickener in recipes and for thickening liquids.

- Salad

The salad is the first meal for acid "refluxers," you should avoid onions and tomatoes, high-fat dressings and cheese.

- Banana

Banana makes a great snack, and at pH 5.6, bananas are great for people with acid reflux. But 1% or 2% of acid refluxers find out that their condition is worsened by bananas. So note this that something that works for most people may not work for you.

- Melon

Melon (pH 6.1) is good for acid reflux. But as for bananas, a small percentage (1% to 2%) of those with acid reflux should avoid it.

- Fennel

Fennel (pH 6.9) is a great food for the acid reflux and it actually seems to improve stomach function. It makes a healthy salad with baby spinach and arugula. Its chicken dishes are great and it makes a fine snack if you really love the taste.

- Chicken and turkey

Poultry is regarded by many as a reflux diet staple. It can be baked, grilled, sautéed or boiled, all you need to do is to remove its high-fat skin.

- Seafood and Fish

Seafood is also another staple of the reflux diet. It must be cooked, baked, or grilled, never fried.

Lobster, shrimp and other shellfish are good on this diet.

- Roots and greens

Green beans, asparagus, broccoli, cauliflower, and other greens are great foods acid reflux. Those on acid reflux diet should simply go for root and green vegetables.

- Celery

This celery has almost no calories because of the high water content, and this a good choice if you have acid reflux. It is also an excellent source of roughage and appetite suppressant.

- Parsley

Over thousands of years now, parsley has started to be used as a medicinal herb to aid digestion. Curly parsley and flat leaf are generally available, and they make a great garnish and seasoning.

- Rice and couscous

Couscous, rice, and bulgur wheat are outstanding foods for acid reflux. They are a source of good carb.

Acid reflux Diet Tips

Your chosen diet plan does not matter, what really matters is the diet plan you choose.

These tips can help to cure acid reflux while you lose weight. While you're losing weight, there are certain foods and drinks that you need to avoid because they trigger your acid reflux. Examples includes spicy foods, coffee, and tomatoes.

After you have lost a considerable amount of weight, you may still eat some of this trigger foods, but it will do you better to totally avoid them for now. They can be gradually introduced after attaining your weight goal.

Avoid chocolate, alcohol, and fried foods. They are a common trigger of acid reflux. By avoiding these foods, calories can be reduced without affecting your good nutrition.

Since you know your daily calorie goal, you can easily divide it into smaller meals over the course of the day. Eating smaller meals frequently will curb overeating and also minimize abdominal pressure. If you prefer the traditional three aquare meals, then keep each meal small and avoid overfilling your stomach.

Do not snack late in the night. Ensure you eat your last meal many hours before bedtime. And while eating, inculcate the habit of eating slowly and leisurely.

CHAPTER FIVE

CONNECTION BETWEEN WEIGHT AND ACID REFLUX

Those who have suffered from acid reflux at one time of their lives could imagine the kind of pain and discomfort the burning sensation does to their chest after overeating or eating the wrong kinds of foods. Going for an acid reflux diet that is devoid of alcohol, caffeine, and spicy foods are usually the first remedy to cure its symptoms. Other measures that should be taken include desisting from smoking, sleeping with an extra pillow, using medications, not wearing tight clothes and avoiding overeating.

However, health experts also discovered that weight loss plays a part in reducing your chances of having acid reflux especially if you were overweight. Therefore, whether you are suffering from an ongoing or occasional form of acid reflux, your weight can play a major factor. Studies also show that most adults who put on extra pounds of weight have high tendency to experience acid reflux but losing weight can be of great relief.

How does overweight and obesity increase the risk of acid reflux?

It's not specifically known how it works, but researchers have it that having an extra fat around the belly puts more pressure on the stomach, thereby causing more fluid to move up into the esophagus.

The sphincter is like a lid that separates the esophagus with the stomach. When more pressure is added to the stomach, the sphincter will be relaxed and opened up to allow acidic fluids from the stomach to make it into the esophagus. Extra weight can also affect the body's ability to empty quickly the stomach contents.

When thin or slim people also overeat, the same scenario plays out as it adds extra pressure on the stomach and sphincter; also pregnancy could also lead to the same scenario.

A Nurse's Health Study research of about 10,000 women found that increase in weight of 10 to 20 pounds corresponds to an increase in acid reflux symptoms. And the symptoms are further increased when obesity sets in. People who are obese have a higher tendency to get acid reflux compared to normal weight people. Loss of weight can reduce acid reflux risk in women to about 40%.

EFFECTS OF YOUR WEIGHT ON ACID REFLUX SYMPTOMS

Acid reflux can affect anyone occasionally but overweight is one of the most common causes. Excess weight increases the pressure on the abdomen thereby causing stomach acid to backflow into the esophagus. Wearing tight-fitted clothing can further heighten the acid reflux symptoms. Whereas losing weight can help reduce its symptoms as it also makes your clothing looser.

Weight gain and other risk factors

As we have previously stated, overweight is one of the biggest risk factor associated with acid reflux. However, there are other temporary reasons for weight gain that can lead to acid reflux such as during pregnancy. But in this case, the symptoms will most likely clear up once a normal weight is attained after delivery.

Acid reflux associated with weight gain can also lead to other health conditions, such as:

- Chest pain
- Asthma
- Sore throat
- A chronic cough and
- Vocal cord tumors

Reduction in the consumption of trigger foods can be of immense benefit to acid reflux in two ways: it can help in the short-term to alleviate symptoms while in the long-term it can help to lose weight.

Weight loss tips

The best way to beat acid reflux is to lose weight. The first step to losing weight is to reduce your daily calorie intake. Reducing your daily intake of high-fat foods can help to reduce your daily calorie intake and also reduce the risk acid reflux. The same also applies to packaged foods, sugars, and other non-nutritive food items.

Another weight loss technique is an exercise, which has proved helpful for people with acid reflux. Taking a walk after a meal helps to burn calories and aids digestion. This habit prevents you from laying down immediately you eat a meal and prevents the risk of stomach acid backflow or leakage. For severe obesity that cannot be resolved with exercise and diet, you might need to go for a weight loss surgery. However, acid reflux is a common side effect of this surgery due to its nature. But it could be well managed in the same way as other lifestyle remedies for acid reflux:

- Eat smaller meals
- Don't eat less than 2 hours before lying down
- Elevate the head of your bed 6-10 inches with a foam wedge
- Eat slowly
- Avoid trigger foods (such as spicy, high-fat foods)

How to Choose a Weight Loss Plan for Acid reflux

It doesn't really matter if the diet is high in fat, high in carbs, or low in protein as the important thing is the daily calorie goals you set which commensurate with your age, gender, level of activity, and weight loss goals. Your daily calorie goal should not be less than 1,200, and not more than 2,400 calories a day. Aim to lose at least 1 to 2 pounds weight per week. Remember, you can lose weight by engaging in physical activity daily as it also reduces your stress levels. Engage in physical activity daily for at least 30 minutes. The physical activity doesn't necessarily need to be running or jogging; it could be as simple as house cleaning, gardening, and walking.

Bottom line

There's a link between acid reflux and excess weight. One of the best lifestyle changes to reduce acid reflux is by losing weight as it also reduces the risk of other health complications. Consult with your gastroenterologist if your acid reflux condition keeps deteriorating despite your best weight loss efforts.

CHAPTER SIX

HOW TO ENSURE SUCCESS ON ACID REFLUX DIET?

It is very important that you seek ways to ensure that your acid reflux diet plan yields its desired result. Your success in adopting the easy ones, but the fast steps will motivate you to move forward and have success with the challenging steps which offer you more impact.

1) You should avoid those tempting trigger foods

The trigger foods lists are fairly well known by most acid reflux experts and physicians. All the following food that aggravate acid reflux should all be avoided if they use to trigger your acid reflux symptoms:

- Fried or fatty foods
- Peppermint and soups
- Most fast foods
- Citrus fruits or spearmint
- Whole milk
- Chocolate creamed
- Tomato paste, onions, garlic and tomatoes
- Tea and coffee
- Carbonated soft drinks
- Spicy or acidic foods

There is an important rule that you need to remember: Everyone is not the same. Which means we are not sure of which food will trigger your symptoms of acid reflux? Most of this trigger food seem to have a very high impact on Acid reflux sufferers, such as raw onions, tomatoes, chocolate and citrus. Nevertheless, smallest possible amounts of these foods or other variations such as dehydrated onions are tolerable ones. It is you only that can determine which foods trigger your symptoms.

I advise that you use trial and error, a food diary or a mobile phone app to keep track of your symptoms against the foods you eat. By passing through a series of test and elimination, you must be able to identify the foods that cause your symptoms. After you have identified it, avoiding these foods, in the end, is the main challenge.

2) Making substitutions and smart food choices

We all need to make choices every day, especially when it has to do with what we eat. These choices can make or mar you and possibly trigger your acid reflux symptoms like never before. You need to make food choices that are smart and you should also show commitment to follow through on the choices you make.

The key to a friendly acid reflux diet is for you to get right substitutions. For example, assuming you love tea, then you need to find ways to avoid or reduce your intake while still satisfying your cravings.

Reduce your caffeine intake; black tea has more caffeine than green tea but it is not in all cases; Herbal is a better choice, and you can even try slippery elm or chamomile, both are known home remedies for acid reflux; you should avoid tea with peppermint or spearmint, both are known triggers.

CHAPTER SEVEN

ACID REFLUX RECIPES

What you eat and how you feel when you eat directly affects your ability to cope with acid reflux. From watching closely what you eat to avoiding your triggers to diet management, they all play critical roles in your acid reflux management.

In this chapter, we would take you through 25 acid reflux recipes that you could enjoy and include in your diet. Here are some delicious and easy to make acid reflux recipes that won't make you feel deprived on your acid reflux diet.

1. Slow cooker chicken and vegetables

This acid reflux recipe contains pineapple, coconut, curry, and turmeric. These combinations blend well and spice up the slow cooker chicken and vegetable recipe.

It's easy to make and delicious – just gently fry the chicken in a frying pan, then leave the rest for the slow cooker to complete.

2. Teriyaki turkey burgers

Even if you are not a big fan of turkey, you will have a change of mind with this recipe. Each bite gives you a burst of flavor as you savor the delicious acid reflux -friendly burgers. Teriyaki turkey burgers are also flavored with ginger and topped with grilled slices of pineapple.

3. Summer Roasted Broccoli Salad

If you want to have a simple but sensational acid reflux friendly dish, then the broccoli salad will cut it for you. This dish has low calories and prepared with some of the most acid reflux friendly spices and healthy coconut oil we have around.

4. Banana Ginger Energy Smoothie

Ingredients

- 2 ripe bananas
- 2 cups of milk
- 2 tablespoons of honey or brown sugar
- ½ cup ice
- 1 cup of yoghurt
- ½ tablespoon of fresh ginger

How to prepare

Put all your ingredients into a blender and blend until smooth. Add sugar to desired taste.

5.   Gala Apple Honeydew Smoothie

Ingredients

- 2 cups of honeydew melon
- 4 tablespoons of freshly peeled Aloe Vera
- 1 peeled Gala apple
- 1/16 tablespoon of lime
- 1 ½ cups of ice
- ¼ tablespoon of salt

How to prepare

Put all your ingredients into a blender and blend until smooth. Press the pulse button on your blender to start your blending process, and then afterward you switch to the high button. At regular intervals, you should stir the mixture to get a smooth consistency.

6. Muesli-Style Oatmeal

Ingredients

- 1 cup of instant oatmeal
- ½ diced banana
- 1 cup of milk
- ½ peeled and diced golden apple
- Pinch of salt
- 2 tablespoon of raisins
- 2 tablespoon of honey or sugar

How to prepare

Mix the ingredients together in a bowl, preferably the evening before, but an hour before too will be just fine. Place it in the refrigerator and add fruit just before serving. You can also add extra milk if the mixture is too thick.

7.   Instant Polenta with Sesame Seeds

Ingredients

- ¾ cup of instant polenta
- 1 tablespoon of sesame seeds
- 3 cups whole milk
- ½ tablespoon of vanilla extract
- 1 tablespoon of orange extract
- 3 tablespoon of brown sugar
- Salt

How to prepare

After boiling the milk add the instant polenta and whip briskly to make it smooth. Then cook until it gets creamy, add the other ingredients such as orange extract, vanilla, sugar, and salt before serving. Serve it in a bowl and sprinkle sesame seeds on the servings.

8 Cauliflower Mac and Cheese

This is a great and healthy recipe for vegetarians suffering from acid reflux. The cauliflower's roasted flavor is really fantastic and a perfect dinner.

The key to its great taste is that the sauce should not be overheated. The eggs should be cooked, but if you allow the sauce to boil, it will possibly thicken. This would affect the texture but won't really affect the flavor. The panko breadcrumb is crunchy and makes it a bit more sophisticated.

The cooking of this recipe will likely take 45 minutes and it can easily be multiplied or cut into two for 2 servings. Leftovers are good. Reheat gently after adding 1 tablespoon of 2% milk per serving.

Ingredients

- 2 tablespoon of olive oil
- 12 ounce of cauliflower

- 6 quarts of water
- 8 ounces of whole wheat
- 2 large eggs
- 1/2 cup of 2 % milk
- 8 ounces of reduced-fat grated white cheddar cheese
- Fresh ground black pepper in sufficient quantity
- 8 Tablespoon of panko breadcrumbs

How to prepare

Place a large frying pan in the oven and preheat to 375°F. Add olive oil to the skillet when hot and afterwards add cauliflower. Turn it well and allow it to roast for about 20 minutes. At an interval of 5 minutes, keep tossing the cauliflower until it is done, then remove and set aside. After this is done, increase the oven's heat to broil.

While cooking the cauliflower, boil your water in a medium stockpot and add your pasta to cook until done. In the process of cooking the pasta, mix the eggs and milk together in a saucepan. Whisk until it becomes smooth. Add salt and the reduced-fat cheddar cheese.

Drain your pasta well after boiling and add you cheese with it in a saucepan to heat at a minimal rate. Keep stirring until the cheese is all creamy and melted. Don't allow it to spend much time on fire and once it begins to get very thick, withdraw from the heat.

Add the roasted cauliflower and fold together gently. Put the Mac and Cheese in oven proof bowls sprinkled with pepper for taste and tablespoons of breadcrumbs.

Place inside the oven for 1 to 2 minutes to lightly toast the breadcrumbs then serve.

9. Cheesecake

The cooking time for this is about 240 Minutes and could be stored for few days, though when fresh it is the better.

Ingredients

- 16 square low-fat graham crackers
- 1 Tablespoon of honey
- 1 large egg white (for crust)
- 8 ounces each of reduced-fat cream and non-fat cream cheese
- 1 cup of sour cream (non-fat)
- 1 cup of cottage cheese
- 1 cup of Granulated Stevia or Splenda
- 1 tablespoon of pure vanilla extract
- 1/4 cup of fresh lemon juice
- 1/4 oz. carton egg substitute
- 1/4 tablespoon salt
- 3 egg whites (for the filling)

You will need to make available a spring form pan along with an 18-inch wide aluminum foil.

How to prepare

Preheat the oven to 300°F. Detach the sides of the springform pan and place the pan bottom on top of two 18-inch square sheets of aluminum foil. Fold the foil edges into a loose cone shape to make it quite easy to be slipped down over the top. Close the sides of the pan around the bottom and then press the foil against the inside of the sides of the pan. The result will be the foil outside the pan on the bottom and inside the pan on the sides.

Pour about 11/2 inches of water into a large roasting pan and place in the oven. Process the cracker in the food processor until they become fine crumbs. Trickle in the honey through the food processor top and then stop the food processor when the honey is well blended with the crumbs.

Gently beat the first egg white in a small mixing bowl until it is lathered. Use a fork to blend the cracker crumbs and the egg whites. Use a spoon to press the crumb mixture down into the bottom of the pan. Then place pan in the oven and cook for ten minutes before removing from the oven.

Leave the coating to cool while you put the other ingredients in a food processor bowl and you keep processing until you achieve a smooth result. Take the remaining egg whites and whisk until they coagulate to form stiff peaks. Fold the mixture in the food processor until they all blend well.

Pour the mixture into the pan and put in a water bath in the oven to bake for about an hour. After this, you switch off the oven, remove the water bath and you then place the cheesecake in the oven without the water bath and leave to cool for about 2 hours. It's best served chilled.

10.   Oven Fried Chicken

The cooking time for this is about 30 Minutes and the leftovers can be preserved for about 2 days without losing its great taste. The oven-fried chicken can go well with a lot of other foods. You can serve with red potato salad, potato vinaigrette salad, healthy French fries, and a host of good combinations.

Ingredients

- 1 Egg
- Chicken breasts
- 5 ounces of plain melba toast
- 1 tablespoon of Dijon mustard
- 1/2 tablespoon of dried oregano
- Oil
- 1/2 tablespoon of ground black pepper
- 1/4 tablespoon of cayenne pepper
- 1/4 tablespoon of garlic powder
- 1 tablespoon of dried thyme
- 1 tablespoon of dried rosemary

- 1/4 tablespoon of salt

How to prepare

Whisk the egg and egg white along with the Dijon mustard until it gets smooth. Place the other ingredients aforementioned into the steel blade fitted food processor and keep processing it until it looks like a breadcrumb.

Preheat oven to 400°F. Put your prepared chicken breast into your egg mixture and immerse your breadcrumbs fresh from the processor also and turn it till they are well coated in the egg mixture.

Use the baking rack to place your chicken in the oven. Allow baking for 3 minutes while you sprinkle oil on the top of your chicken breast. Leave it for another 5 minutes then you turn. Spray the other side with oil lightly and bake for 6 more minutes. This recipe works well with any part of the chicken.

11.   Calm Carrot Salad

Ingredients

- Carrots
- Tablespoon of olive oil
- Tablespoon of dried oregano
- ¼ lb. mesclun greens
- Tablespoon of brown sugar
- Tablespoon of raisins
- Tablespoon of orange juice
- ¼ Tablespoon of salt

How to prepare

Mix the ingredients together in a bowl and allow it to settle for about 5 minutes. Pour the mixture over the blended and diced carrots and mix thoroughly. Taste and season with extra salt if needed. It should be served over mesclun leaves.

12.   Black Bean and Cilantro Soup

Ingredients

- 8 oz of canned black beans
- ½ cup of fresh cilantro
- a pint of chicken stock
- 1 tablespoon of nonfat sour cream
- Salt

How to prepare

Boil the chicken stock and cook on a low heat for about 30 minutes along with your beans, cilantro, and salt. After cooking, blend with a hand blender to get your desired consistency. Put the right quantity of seasoning and serve garnished with cilantro and 1 tablespoon of non-fat sour cream.

13.　　Flavorful Cantaloupe Gazpacho

Ingredients

- 2 cups of cantaloupe
- Tablespoon of port wine
- Tablespoon of brown sugar
- Fine-grated nutmeg

How to prepare

Mix the ingredients together and freeze for about
4 hours. Then you blend it
and finish it with nutmeg dust. It could be served
immediately with a small
cup.

14.　　Creamy Hummus

Ingredients

- Canned chickpeas

- 1 cup of chicken stock
- Tablespoon of olive oil
- ¼ tablespoon of sesame oil
- ½ tablespoon of salt

How to prepare

Put your canned chickpeas into a food processor and add your other ingredients to it. Keep processing until it becomes smooth. Add more chicken. stock as you will need. It should be served cold and goes well with foods like flatbread or oven-toasted corn chips.

15. Watermelon and Ginger Granite

Ingredients

- 3 cups of blended watermelon juice
- Water
- 1 tablespoon of fresh ginger

- 1 pinch of ground nutmeg
- ½ cup honey
- 1 whole clove
- ½ tablespoon of lemon zest
- 1 tsp. salt

How to prepare

Gather your ingredients, boil it together, and allow cooling before you drain. Add this cooked mixture to the blended watermelon juice. Place the resulting juice in a freezer for about 3 hours then you stir every 15 minutes.

16.   Lentil and Chickpea Soup

The cooking time for this recipe takes about 75 minutes, which is different from the time it takes to soak the chickpeas and lentils. This recipe can be used multiple times and it still looks better the next day.

Ingredients

- 2 quarts of water
- 4 ounces of dried lentils
- 3 bay leaves
- 2 tablespoon of olive oil
- Vegetable stock
- 4 ounces of diced celery
- Fresh ground black pepper
- 4 ounces of peeled and diced carrots
- 1/4 tablespoon of salt

How to prepare

Soak your lentils and chickpeas in water for at least 10 hours. After 10 hours, you should drain and rinse. Pour the olive oil into a large saucepan and apply medium-high heat. Add your celery and leave to cook for about 4 minutes until it becomes slightly luminous. After 4 minutes, you should also add your carrots to cook for about 3 minutes. At every time you add a new ingredient, remember to stir vigorously. Add the lentils, chickpeas, vegetable stock, and bay leaves. Allow them to all simmer together for about 45 minutes on a medium-low heat. Lastly, put the salt and pepper and allow them to all simmer for extra 15 minutes. Allow it to cool down before serving.

17.   Quick Banana Sorbet

Ingredients

- 3 bananas, peeled
- Tablespoon of honey
- Cups of ice
- Tablespoon of ginger
- 1/8 tablespoon of ground cardamom
- ¼ tablespoon of salt

How to prepare

Blend your ingredients together until it becomes smooth and then add ice and blend until it gets creamy. You can either preserve it in the freezer or serve immediately.

18.   Mushroom Salad

The estimated time needed to cook this recipe is just 30 minutes and it can be multiplied. You won't really enjoy this recipe if you have a leftover so it's often advised that you only prepare what you can finish within 24 hours.

Ingredients

- 8 ounces of sliced mushrooms
- Romaine lettuce leaf
- 2 tablespoon of reduced fat sour cream
- 1 tablespoon of olive oil
- 2 tablespoon of coarse ground mustard
- Ground black pepper

- 2 tablespoon of 2% milk
- 1/2 tablespoon of fresh orange
- 2 tablespoon of vinegar
- 1/8 tablespoon of salt to taste

Mix all the ingredients together and chill. Then slice the mushrooms thinly with it when you are done. Serve along with the romaine leaf.

19.   Cranberry Bacon Brussels sprouts

This recipe cooking time is going to take 30 minutes and it can be multiplied and preserved in the refrigerated for about 4-5 days.

Ingredients

- Fresh Brussels sprouts
- 2 tablespoon of dried sweetened cranberries
- 2 ounces of finely minced bacon

- Fresh ground black pepper to taste

How to prepare

Trim the fresh Brussels sprouts stems and then cut into thin slices while you do away with any of the tough core. Place the finely-minced bacon in a large pot and heat. Watch the bacon closely and ensure to adjust the heat to prevent it from burning or cooking to fast. After about 10 minutes, add your cranberries and leave to cook for 5 minutes. Then you add your pepper and brussels sprouts and leave to simmer for about 5 minutes.

20.   Chinese Chicken Salad

This recipe will take about 45 minutes to cook and it can be kept for 24 hours to avoid it losing its savor.

Ingredients

- 3 quarts of water

- 8 oz of whole wheat
- 2 tablespoon of sesame oil
- 4 oz of thinly sliced mushrooms
- spray oil
- 1/4 cup of slivered almonds
- 16 oz of chicken breast
- 1 tablespoon of low-sodium soy sauce
- 8 oz of thinly sliced cabbage
- 8 oz of thinly sliced carrots
- 4 ounces of snow peas
- 3 tablespoon of hoisin sauce
- 2 tablespoon of rice vinegar
- 2 tablespoon of pineapple juice
- Mandarin oranges

You can as well include the sesame seeds

How to prepare

Heat your water in a medium stockpot. Allow the water to boil before adding your udon noodles, leave it for about 6-8 minutes to cook properly, and then you drain off excess water, and place the well-drained noodles in a large mixing bowl. Add sesame oil and stir until it's thoroughly mixed. Then you put in the refrigerator.

Put water in a large non-stick skillet and adjust to the medium heat. Sprinkle little oil and add sliced mushrooms. Keep turning the mushrooms in the oil until they begin to brown. At this stage, you should add your almonds and keep stirring frequently until the almonds color turns light brown. Then you remove and set aside.

Set your oven temperature to 375°F and place a large skillet on it. Sprinkle oil on the pan and add your prepared chicken breasts. Allow cooking for 8 minutes before turning the chicken to the other side. Add your soy sauce and leave to cook for an about 5 more minutes. By then, your chicken should be well cooked. Next, you cut the chicken into 1/4 inch strips.

By then you should have also prepared your hoisin sauce mixed together with the rice vinegar, while you also prepare your pineapple juice.

Allow the chicken to cool then you fold it alongside the udon noodles, carrots, cabbage, snow peas and dressing. Its serving should be accompanied with the mushroom and almond mixture not leaving out the mandarin oranges. Some might also prefer to garnish it with sesame seeds, it's cool.

21.   Roasted Beet and Fennel Salad

The estimated cooking time is 90 minutes. The recipe can last for about 72 hours while retaining its flavor. Simply ensure it's kept in the refrigerator.

Ingredients

- 2 large beets
- 1 lb of fresh fennel
- 1/2 tablespoon of ground cumin
- 1 ounce of feta cheese
- 1 tablespoon of olive oil
- fresh ground black pepper
- 1/4 tablespoon of salt

How to prepare

Preheat the oven to 375°F. Trim off the stem and tip of the beets. Ensure its well-scrubbed and neatly wrapped in aluminum foil. Place your well-cut beets into the oven and allow it to roast for 45 minutes. Then you remove and allow it to cool.

Prepare your fennel too by removing the leafy ends from the fennel and cutting off any tough stalk. Then slice thinly. Pour your olive oil into a small pan and apply medium heat. Add your thinly sliced fennel and cook for about 15 minutes with occasional stirring.

Remove and allow cooling. Detach the beets from the aluminum foil and peel off the skin after which you should cut into 1/2 inch cubes. Mix the beets together with the fennel, ground cumin, crumbled feta, black pepper and add salt to taste.

22.   Rosemary Turkey Skewers

This delicious recipe will take about 30 minutes to cook. This recipe can also be multiplied. This recipe tastes good even when leftover for several days. The skewers can even be prepared 48 hours in advance and kept in the refrigerator.

It could be served along with other wonderful delicacies such as wild rice or cranberry glaze. It could also be served alongside veggies for veggies lovers such as the sautéed spinach or minted carrots.

Ingredients

- 16 ounces of turkey breast
- 2 tablespoon of extra virgin olive oil
- 2 tablespoon of fresh rosemary
- 1/2 tablespoon of salt
- Fresh ground black pepper
- Olive oil

How to prepare

Slice the turkey into thin strips according to your servings. Place the turkey strips on wooden skewers. Ensure that each skewer has two strips. Put the turkey skewers in a bag. Add your other ingredients, fresh rosemary, olive oil, pepper, and salt. Mix them thoroughly well and close the bag. It should be placed in the refrigerator overnight.

When you want to serve it, moderately heat a frying pan, sprinkle with olive oil and add the skewers. Leave to cook for about 5 minutes before you turn. Keep turning until it spends at least 15 minutes on fire before you remove and serve.

23.   Butternut Squash Soup

The estimated cooking time for this recipe is 60 Minutes. You can enjoy the leftovers from this recipe and it can be multiplied by 2, 3, 4. Serve with whole wheat, semi-soft goat cheese, and fennel salad.

Ingredients

- 2 cups of water
- 2 lbs of butternut squash
- 1/2 tablespoon of salt
- Fresh ground black pepper
- 1/2 tablespoon of dried thyme leaves
- 1/8 tablespoon of ground nutmeg
- Water

How to prepare

Put water into a large saucepan over high heat and well fitted with a steamer basket. Steam along with the cubed squash for about 20- 30 minutes.

Allow the squash to cool before pouring it into the steaming water left at the bottom of the saucepan. Blend the squash and water well until it gives a smooth mixture. Include your other ingredients into the pan that is on the fire with a low heat. Gently reheat the soup. Add more water until you get your desired quantity.

24.   Cannellini Bean Soup

The cooking time for this recipe is 30 minutes (if you are using canned beans, but if you are using dried beans it will be up to 90 minutes).

This recipe can be multiplied and divisible by 2. You will enjoy this recipe better when served chilled. It can be kept in the refrigerator for about 72 hours without it losing its taste.

You can serve it alongside whole grain and Waldorf salad or roasted beet and fennel salad.

Ingredients

- Cannellini beans
- 3 quarts of water
- 1 tablespoon of olive oil
- 1 large and diced white onion
- Fresh ground black pepper
- 2 cups of vegetable broth
- 2 ribs of minced celery
- 2 cloves of minced garlic
- 2 tablespoon of fresh oregano
- 1/4 tablespoon of salt

How to prepare

If you are using dry beans, pour it in a large pot covered with water. Allow it to soak overnight. The next day, drain the beans and cover with water and out in the fire with a medium-high heat. When it starts to boil, reduce the heat to a simmer. Give it about 60min while you ensure the beans soften well.

Drain the water from the beans and remove from the fire. Rinse the pot as you pour the olive oil into it with a medium heat also. Include your onions and garlic. Cook slowly until the onions color changes to translucent. Put the beans back into the pot and stir it well to mix. Then include your chicken stock with salt to taste. Allow cooking for another 10 minutes while you stir occasionally. Include your other ingredients and cook for another extra 20 minutes.

Then use your blender to blend the soup in batches until you get your desired texture. You may serve this soup hot or chilled.

25. Chicken and Black-Eyed Pea Soup

The estimated cooking time for this meal is about 60 Minutes. You can preserve this recipe at its best quality for up to 48 hours. It can be served with a whole lot of delicious recipes such as the cornbread muffins.

Ingredients

- 1 lb of chicken thighs
- 2 tablespoon of dried sage
- 1/2 tablespoon of dried thyme
- 8 ounces of fresh spinach
- Tablespoon of olive oil
- 1 large red onion
- 3 cups of low sodium chicken or vegetable broth
- Celery
- Black-eyed peas
- 1/2 tablespoon of salt
- Fresh ground black pepper

How to prepare

Heat the olive oil over medium heat in a large saucepan. Add the celery and onions while you stir frequently to cook for about 7 minutes when the onions start to soften.

Add the chicken thighs, sage, thyme, and cook, stirring frequently until the chicken is lightly browned – about 5 – 7 minutes.

Include your other ingredients such as chicken stock, salt, pepper, black-eyed peas and of course water. Increase the intensity of the heat while you reduce it when you notice that the soup has started boiling. This will allow the soup to simmer. Allow the cooking to last for about 40 minutes, while you stir occasionally.

When you want to serve, put 2-ounce spinach at the bottom of the bowl while you pour two cups of soup on top of it.

There is several other acid reflux recipe that you can also enjoy and combine to give you a great diet and effectively eliminate the symptoms associated with acid reflux.

CONCLUSION

This nutritional guide ensures you have adequate knowledge of what acid reflux is and how you can effectively tackle or guide it. If you only skimmed through to get here, I would advise that you go back to the chapters above and learn some important facts about acid reflux.

From your lifestyle changes to your triggers to your weight loss, you can start saying goodbye to your acid reflux and start living a more hearty and healthy life.

----- *BILL HILLON*

If you enjoyed this book or benefited from it in any way, then I would greatly appreciate if you would be kind enough to leave a review for this book on Amazon.

Please click below link to leave a review on Amazon.com.

https://www.amazon.com/review/create-review?asin=B079VXVFD5#

Thank You.

Check Out Other Books

Go here to check out other related books that might interest you:

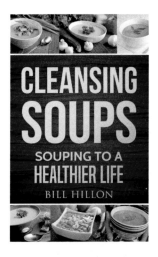

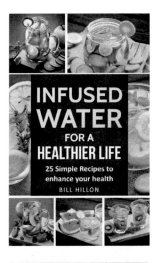

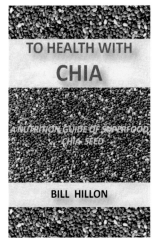

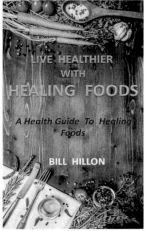

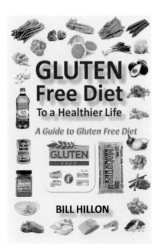

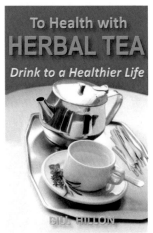

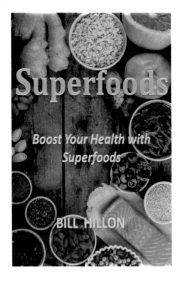

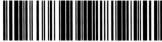

77764069R00044

Made in the USA
Middletown, DE
25 June 2018